I0470982

Health Disclaimer

Dr. Susan Plank provides scientific information on the health aspects of dietary factors and supplements, foods, and beverages for the general public. This information is made available with the understanding that the author is not providing medical, psychological, or nutritional counseling services in this book. The information should not be used in place of a consultation with a competent health care or nutrition professional.

The information on dietary factors and supplements, foods, and beverages contained in this publication does not cover all possible uses, actions, precautions, side effects, and interactions. It is not intended as nutritional or medical advice for individual problems. Liability for individual actions or omissions based upon the contents of this publication is expressly disclaimed.

CONTENTS

PREFACE

I am a traumatic brain injury (TBI) survivor. I never imagined I would be writing a book on improving life after brain injury. I was thrilled to be a chiropractor, helping address muscular and structural symptoms in my clients. I dabbled in preventive healthcare; watch what you eat, exercise, the usual advice a healthcare provider gives.

In 2006 I volunteered as part of a church mission trip after Hurricane Katrina. While in Slidell, Louisiana I fell from a ladder while mucking out a devastated house. I landed on my head.

I struggled to be accurately diagnosed, and I struggled to get treatment to feel whole again. It was the beginning of a long journey, a never ending journey.

As my rehab funding was running out and the affects of my deficits were growing, I began scouring books, journals, and the internet, anything that could potentially help me to improve cognitively. I was losing the life I had known; the life I had worked for and I couldn't accept my situation.

Adjusting to life as a survivor was not easy. My life was familiar but new, not mine, not as I'd known mine to be. My misfiring synapses; forgotten name, misspoken word, or burst of anger caught me off guard; and those around me. As a survivor, I learned that vulnerability was a constant.

As a result of my search for improvement, I started taking a supplement which improved my cognitive endurance quickly. Previously, I could only work for about a 20 minute stretch productively. Taking a break meant forgetting where I was; what I was working on and continuing meant cognitive overload, confusion, anger, tears and usually exhaustion. After eight months I could only work 20 minutes at a time and within that month I jumped to 40 continuous focused minutes. The supplement worked, I was on fire!

I realized I needed physical stamina as well as cognitive endurance. As my physical symptoms improved with the help of chiropractic, yoga and physical therapy I started to exercise. It felt good to get my heart pumping but the increase in exertion brought back some of my vertigo; I had to learn to modify my behavior. I had to set limits. This was new to me; pre-injury I could stay up late, handle stress better and go-go-go. Life was different now.

Time has passed and I have continually worked at improving various aspects of my health. It has taken seven years for me to settle into the person I am now. To become comfortable with whom I am; what I can do and what I might be capable of.

I have been a presenter at the Pennsylvania Brain Injury Association (PABIA.org) conferences on nutritional and complementary medicine. I have spoken at brain injury support groups and symposiums on the cognitive benefits of eating well and taking better care of you. I have become a health consultant, educating and helping others to make positive changes in their health. I still enjoy being a chiropractor but I love writing, presenting and working with my nutritional clients.

This manual is designed to guide you to choices that may help you to improve your cognition, memory, energy and stamina. The framework is supplied but YOU have to put in the effort and time.

My life is more fulfilling than I'd imagined possible and while I am anxious to see what's next, I'll warn you, I still experience synaptic misfires. I still feel mildly embarrassed and vulnerable but I don't let it be a road block to my goals. Don't allow frustration to hinder you. Don't lose sight of the long term goal, improving your cognitive health so you feel better mentally and physically.

I am thankful for those who have continually believed in me, who helped guide and support me in the good times and the not so good times.

I have been truly blessed by: God, Uni, Cindy, Steve and Mom (I miss you every day!)

I also would like to thank all the friends and caregivers that showed me patience and compassion. I couldn't have done it without you: Becky, Dottie, Gary, Mary Lou, Lynne, Mick, Jeff, Linda, and Sandra.

Susan Plank, D.C.

1

MAKING GOOD CHOICES: HOW TO CHANGE YOUR HABITS

Have you heard of the mind-body connection? It's the reason anxiety or nervousness can cause butterflies in your stomach. It's a physical manifestation of our emotions and is perfectly normal.

After we experience an emotion we typically respond with a behavior. Some behaviors are healthy and acceptable while other behaviors can be self destructive.

In order to change our habits we need to look at our feelings, our emotional and physical needs, our behaviors and the consequences of our habits or behaviors.

Let me say, I'm not a psychologist. I only want you to be aware of the process of how our habits and behaviors are formed. I believe strongly that to change one has to understand fully what is happening and why it is happening.

Let's look at a couple examples:

A mom is lonely. Her son and husband don't seem to listen or pay attention to her any more. Every time she walks past the candy bowl on the counter she's eating two or three chocolates. She's gained fifteen pounds in the last three months.

Let's take a closer look:

The mom is lonely (emotion). She needs attention, love or to feel valued (emotional need). She eats chocolate (behavior). Result is she gains weight (consequence).

Another example:

A lackadaisical teenage boy wants more respect from his parents; they are constantly nagging him about cleaning his room, doing chores and getting into college. After a fight with them he leaves the house in anger one night, picks up his friend and they drive to a party. His friend prompts him to have a few beers, the teenager, wanting to fit in, obliges. He's having fun; he drinks more trying to forget the argument with parents. Driving home that night his erratic driving causes a terrible accident.

Let's take a closer look:

The boy is angry (emotion). He wants respect (emotional need). He drinks beer and drives (behavior). He hurts himself and his friend (consequence).

What are your feelings, needs and behaviors? Do you have chocolate eating moments? Angry out bursts? Do you have emotional triggers that are causing poor behavior choices? You can change. I know you can.

After my brain injury my dizziness was terrible. I'd get nauseous and was losing weight. My physical therapist had given me exercises to help my vertigo but I didn't make time to do them. They didn't seem important. Time went by and no improvement, still dizzy, I grew frustrated that therapy was a waste of time. I allowed myself to be a victim to my injury.

When I started doing my vestibular exercises I started to improve. I suffered for months because I was angry and depressed about how much I had lost (and was losing) from my brain injury that my emotions held me back and became part of the problem. I was allowing myself to remain dizzy!

Challenge yourself to figure what your patterns are and H-A-L-T them. When you reach for another donut; when you won't get off the couch to exercise; when you yell at your caregiver; if you think a drink will make you feel better, I want you to H-A-L-T and ask yourself these four questions.

1. **H**:   Are you **H**ungry?
2. **A**:   Are you **A**ngry?
3. **L**:   Are you **L**onely?
4. **T**:   Are you **T**ired?

The answers to these four physical-emotional questions may be holding you back; blocking your potential. Keeping you from the person you can become. Let's look closer at the four physical-emotional triggers.

1. **H**: Are you hungry? If you answer yes, you might actually be hungry, then you can simply go make yourself something healthy to eat and that will fix your physical state of hunger. But if we look at "Are you hungry?" emotionally, then we might look at this question as "Are you hungry for more?" or "What's missing in your life?" You may be emotionally hungry.

That's usually when trouble starts, when we deal with our anger inappropriately. Look a little deeper and see what you are hungry for; it might be a hunger food won't satisfy!

2. **A**: Are you angry? It's normal to feel angry, but how do you show it? That's usually when trouble starts, do we deal with our anger appropriately.

Anger can start with resentment. Since your injury do you feel as if you are being treated like a child? Are you annoyed or aggravated by the same situations over and over? For example, as a survivor are you having difficulty with a task that used to come easily before your injury? You may resent your injury or those trying to help you and resentment can lead to anger.

If not dealt with properly, anger can be destructive. We can turn it inward, hurting ourselves, or we can lash out with words and actions and hurt others.

Are you angry? Do you know why? Cognitive behavioral therapy is a specific psychotherapy approach designed to help identify the triggering emotions and negative thoughts that cause our anger to become hurtful and destructive. Consider getting help from a licensed therapist, they will be able to help you. Other techniques such as relaxation, deep breathing and mindfulness can also be helpful.

3. **L:** Are you lonely? Are you depressed or possibly isolating yourself? You may be lacking the companionship you desire. Try

to reach out to family or friends. Definitely, consider seeing a therapist to help you problem solve through loneliness. Contact a local brain injury support group. Others are going through the same struggles that you are experiencing. You are NOT alone.

Have you lost friends, your spouse or significant other since your injury? Have you been able to develop new friendships? Is it possible you hunger for friends, for compassion, for a sense of belonging?

4. **T**: Are you tired? Sounds simple, just nap or get some sleep. Eighty four percent of brain injury survivors report having difficulty sleeping. As a survivor your judgment may be impaired and lack of sleep will exacerbate your decision making. Set boundaries, pace yourself; talk with your cognitive therapy team about your physical and cognitive limits. When you're cognitively tired everything becomes more difficult. Make sure you have realistic,

achievable goals and that you are using appropriate time management strategies.

After my injury, if I allowed myself to become mentally or physically fatigued, my anger would rise. I could become nasty in an instant, I felt terrible after the words were spoken but had difficulty holding my tongue. I had to find what my emotional and physical limits were and share that with my family, friends and therapists. I had to know my limits before I could ask others to respect my limits.

2

YOUR WEIGHT CAN AFFECT YOUR BRAIN

Did you know being overweight is a risk factor in developing dementia and in decreasing your cognitive abilities? Middle aged individuals (30-50) and older individuals (60+) are at greater risk of cognitive impairment due to being overweight. Just an eight to ten percent decrease in your weight has been shown to improve physical strength and cognition, especially processing speed.

Weight gain can be quick after suffering a brain injury. Research of weight gain among children that had suffered a traumatic brain injury (TBI) was quick and excessive. Obesity after TBI can also be related to a decrease in growth hormone and pituitary changes, especially in children. Other factors associated with an increased weight gain after TBI include mobility restrictions, being male and being older.

A lower cognitive performance earlier in life can be a factor in increased weight gain throughout life. Obesity does lead to other health factors. Research has shown that obesity in addition to other medical issues such as diabetes and hypertension can be very detrimental to cognitive abilities. Obesity by itself is a factor in developing Type 2 diabetes, increased cholesterol levels, degenerative arthritis, heart disease, hypertension, stroke and many forms of cancer.

After suffering my brain injury my motto is *Protect What I Have.* In other words I know my brain suffered some damage when I fell, so now I need to make good choices to help protect the brain cells I have and prevent further damage!

What should you weigh? There are multiple ways to determine your optimal weight. One method is to determine your Ideal Body Weight (IBW). This method has been primarily used by the insurance industry over the years when writing life insurance policies. It is a simple chart format (See Figure 1). Find your height in the left hand column and appropriate sex in the top of the columns and

Male		Female	
Height	**Ideal Weight**	**Height**	**Ideal Weight**
4' 10"	85 - 103 lbs.	4' 10"	81 - 99 lbs.
4' 11"	90 - 110 lbs.	4' 11"	86 - 105 lbs.
5' 0"	95 - 117 lbs.	5' 0"	90 - 110 lbs.
5' 1"	101 - 123 lbs.	5' 1"	95 - 116 lbs.
5' 2"	106 - 130 lbs.	5' 2"	99 - 121 lbs.
5' 3"	112 - 136 lbs.	5' 3"	104 - 127 lbs.
5' 4"	117 - 143 lbs.	5' 4"	108 - 132 lbs.
5' 5"	122 - 150 lbs.	5' 5"	113 - 138 lbs.
5' 6"	128 - 156 lbs.	5' 6"	117 - 143 lbs.
5' 7"	133 - 163 lbs.	5' 7"	122 - 149 lbs.
5' 8"	139 - 169 lbs.	5' 8"	126 - 154 lbs.
5' 9"	144 - 176 lbs.	5' 9"	131 - 160 lbs.
5' 10"	149 - 183 lbs.	5' 10"	135 - 165 lbs.
5' 11"	155 - 189 lbs.	5' 11"	140 - 171 lbs.
6' 0"	160 - 196 lbs.	6' 0"	144 - 176 lbs.
6' 1"	166 - 202 lbs.	6' 1"	149 - 182 lbs.
6' 2"	171 - 209 lbs.	6' 2"	153 - 187 lbs.
6' 3"	176 - 216 lbs.	6' 3"	158 - 193 lbs.

Figure 1. Ideal Body Weight: Find your height under the appropriate gender column. Your acceptable weight range is listed beside your height.

where the two intersect is your Ideal Body Weight. Your IBW is given as an acceptable weight range but it is not necessarily indicative of your overall health.

Percent body fat is another method of determining a satisfactory weight (See Figure 2). It is reflective of how much fat you are carrying; it is the total weight of your fat divided by your total weight. Determining your total fat is the key to the equation.

Fitness Level	Men	Women
Essential Body Fat	3-5%	10-16%
Pro Athletes	6-13%	14-20%
A Fit Individual	14-17%	21-24%
Average	18-24%	25-31%
Unfit/Obese	25%+	32%+

Figure 2. Percent body fat and expected fitness levels.

Each of us has essential body fat and stored body fat. Essential fat is necessary to sustaining life and reproductive functions. Women have a higher acceptable essential body fat percentage than men, for women 10-16% is considered normal and for men 3-5%.

Stored body fat accumulates around organs, and in the abdomen and chest. Stored body fat compresses the organs and can block blood flow. Stored body fat is detrimental to your health.

Percent body fat is a measure of fitness; it does not rely on height or weight measurements. It is reflective of the composition of an individual. There is some controversy as to whether a specific body fat percentage is better for one's health.

 Although, not economical, the most accurate way to determine percent body fat is by the water displacement method. Other ways to directly measure percent body fat are by bioelectrical impedance (requiring a specialized scale) and the use of calipers to measure body skin folds.

The equation to calculate your percent body fat is complex. If you are interested in knowing your percent body fat, I would recommend a quick search online. There are many online sites that allow you to enter your body measurements and will calculate your percent body fat for you!

The best method to determine your optimal weight is the Body Mass Index or BMI. BMI does not directly measure body fat stores but the BMI chart (See Figure 3) has proven to be accurate in determining body fat. It is inexpensive, can be used by women or men and is an excellent screening tool in determining potential weight and associated health problems.

FOOD IS FUEL

Food supplies us with vitamins and nutrients we need to function optimally. We also consume food and drink for emotional reasons. Birthdays, pay raises and Happy Hours are ways we celebrate with food and drink. Occasional excesses are understandable but will add weight.

Is dieting the answer? No. For lasting success you need to change your outlook, change your habits. Change the way you look at food, take an honest look at what you are eating and drinking, remember food is fuel to your body. Cupcakes, pizza, burgers and soda are not fueling your body. If you continue to eat these types of food, you are making the choice to hurt your health, *YOU* are making yourself sick!

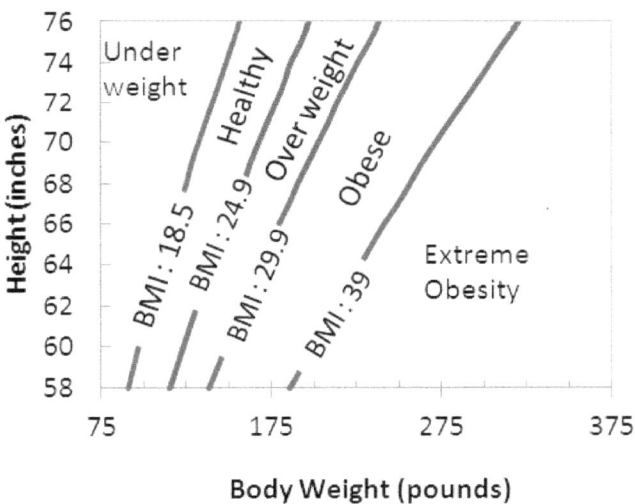

Figure 3. Body mass index (BMI) chart for use in adults over 20 years of age. Underweight: Less than 18.5. Ideal: 18.5-24.9. Overweight: 25-29.9. Very Overweight/Obese: Greater than 30.

HOW MUCH EXERCISE DO YOU HAVE TO DO TO EAT THE WAY YOU WANT TO?

Did you know a glazed donut has 190 calories? A plain cheeseburger has 300 calories. You may think this doesn't sound like much but do you know you'd have to walk an hour to burn off the donut and 90 minutes to burn off the cheeseburger. Are you willing to do that? Figure 4 shows typical American food choices and the number of calories they contain. Figure 5 shows various forms of exercise and the number of calories each would burn. The longer an exercise can be sustained the better the body's ability to burn calories.

To lose weight you need to make better food fuel choices and *get moving* to burn off the stored fat!

FOOD	NUMBER OF CALORIES
APPLE	72
PEAR	96
SNICKERS™ CANDY BAR	280
PEPPERONI PIZZA-2 SLICES	500
CHEESEBURGER	300
FRIES-SMALL	230
SODA-EIGHT OUNCES	94

Figure 4. Typical foods and their caloric values.

EXERCISE	NUMBER OF CALORIES BURNED
WALK- 20 MINUTES	65
WALK- 60 MINUTES	196
PUSH UP - 1 MINUTE	10
JUMPING JACKS- 1 MINUTE	11
BICYCLING-30 MINUTES EASY	157

Figure 5. Typical exercises and their caloric expenditures.

3

HIGH POTENCY MULTIVITAMIN

Good nutrition and regular exercise are integral to attaining and maintaining good physical and emotional health. Try to eat a healthy and varied diet, especially rich in vibrant colored fruits and vegetables and lower fat proteins. Unfortunately, it is impossible to eat a balanced diet all the time. That's when supplementation can be beneficial. Supplements won't make up for a lousy diet but can add to a good one.

Recent research has shown a good quality multivitamin to be beneficial for older men, especially in relation to the risk of developing cancer. Also, taking a multivitamin can ensure adequate nutrient intake to prevent chronic disease.

When looking for a good multivitamin and mineral supplement read the manufacturing label on the package to insure adequate levels of the recommended daily allowance (RDA) of vitamins. Adequate vitamins and minerals are necessary to maintain your energy and vitality (See Figure 6).

In nutritional terms, the RDA is the minimum amount needed of a vitamin or mineral to maintain a minimum of health. If you are recovering from a brain injury, another condition or surgery, leading an active life or fighting a cold you probably need more nutrients than are in your multivitamin. That's why they are called supplements, to supplement your healthy diet.

Multivitamin supplements tout specific focuses; Men 50+, Energy Support, Menopausal Woman Formula, etc. I haven't found a "broken brain" multivitamin yet but soon we may have one!

A note of caution some vitamins advertised as energy, weight loss or metabolism boosting vitamins contain caffeine or herbs that contain caffeine. If you are sensitive to caffeine and it makes you jittery, read the ingredient label cautiously. Herbs such as guarana, kola nut or yerba mate contain caffeine. Ma huang is a traditional Chinese herb that contains ephedra and acts as a stimulant, increasing the heart rate like caffeine does. Also, like caffeine, these herbs can be habit forming, causing a headache or feeling of uneasiness when removed from your diet.

I'd also advise you to take your vitamins with breakfast but not after lunch as the energy that the B vitamins provide may keep you awake at night. As brain injury survivors we need good quality sleep. We'll see later why sleep is important to the brain.

VITAMIN	RDA MALES*	RDA FEMALES*	UNITS
VITAMIN A**	3000	2333	IU
50% AS BETA-CAROTENE			IU
B1, THIAMINE	1.2	1.1	MG
B2, RIBOFLAVIN	1.3	1.1	MG
B3, NIACIN	16	14	MG
B6, PYRIDOXINE	1.3	1.3	MG
B12	2.4	2.4	MCG
FOLIC ACID/FOLATE	400	400	MCG
VITAMIN C	90	75	MG
VITAMIN D	600	600	IU
VITAMIN E	22.5	22.5	IU

Figure 6. Recommended daily allowance (RDA).

*for Adults 19 yrs old and older
**Vitamin A: Most multivitamins contain 5000IU of Vitamin A. Consider a multivitamin that contains a maximum of 2500 IU of Vitamin A and also 2500 IU of Beta-Carotene to avoid any Vitamin A toxicity.

RDA source: Office of Dietary Supplements; National Institutes of Health; Food and Nutrition Board; Institute of Medicine; Linus Pauling Institute.

4

FATTY ACIDS and FISH OIL

Essential fatty acids (EFA) are required by the body but the body is not able to make them, therefore, EFA's must be consumed in the diet. EFA's have many functions, they are important in many biologic pathways and to insure the body works optimally. Fatty acids, because of their name, should not be negatively confused with fat.

Omega-3 and omega-6 are the most widely known fatty acids. The relationship and balance of omega-3 to omega-6 fatty acids in the body control the biologic function they exhibit on the body. The balance of omega-3 and omega-6 affects cellular signaling, mood and behavior. An imbalance between omega-3 and omega-6 can cause inflammatory conditions and also changes in mood and behavior.

Plant sources of essential fatty acids are Linoleic Acid (LA), an omega-6 fatty acid; it is found in plant oils such as safflower oil and corn oil. Alpha-Linolenic Acid (ALA), an omega-3 essential fatty acid, is found in flaxseed oil and walnuts.

Cold deep water fish are the best sources of omega-3 fatty acids. Fish such as herring, salmon, krill and anchovy offer some of the highest amounts of omega-3 fatty acids. Omega-3 fatty acids are found in the form of eicosapentaenoic acid (EPA) and docosahexaenoic acid (DHA). In high quality fish oil supplements the label should distinguish the amount of EPA and DHA contained per serving.

DHA, found in fish oil, is the most prominent fatty acid in the brain and it appears to be protective against cognitive decline, dementia and Alzheimer's disease. Research has shown those individuals that consume oily fish three times a week had the least chance of developing any form of dementia including Alzheimer's disease.

The typical American diet is much higher in omega-6 than omega-3 fatty acids. Typically the omega-6 oils are the oils in which our foods are cooked and deep fried. This is believed to be a major consideration in the United States' higher incidence of inflammation and chronic diseases such as cardiovascular disease, vision problems, dementia and osteoporosis. Scientific research suggests that increasing omega-3 fatty acids in the diet would reduce the incidence of heart disease.

It is believed that wild caught fish has a greater level of omega-3 than farm raised fish. Farm raised fish's diet consists mostly of grain vs. wild caught fish consisting of algae, plankton and other smaller fish. While wild caught fish is more expensive, if it's not consistently in your budget, I recommend taking fish oil supplements when eating your farm raised fish.

When looking for a fish oil supplement compare the EPA and DHA levels from the label to insure good quality. Omega-3 fatty acids are more efficiently absorbed with meals and spreading your daily intake throughout the day helps ensure proper absorption.

Standard omega-3 dosage is 1000mg/day, which is equivalent to one gram. Research has shown omega-3 fatty acids supplementation in TBI induced rats showed improvement in synaptic plasticity, cognition and may prevent disability following TBI. Therapeutic dosage of three g/day (3000 mg/d) has shown to be beneficial for brain injury survivors. Fish oil supplements may contain a small amount of vitamin E as a preservative.

Larger predatory fish can have higher levels of mercury. For this reason eliminate or limit consumption of shark, swordfish, king mackerel, golden bass or snapper. Limit canned tuna to six ounces per week. The most commonly consumed fish that are low in mercury include shrimp, salmon, catfish and Pollock.

Precautions: While the consumption of fish and utilization of fish oil supplements can be very beneficial, there has been no safety limits established for pregnant or lactating women. Potential for adverse affects are low but consumers of fish oil should be cautious for: digestive upset, loose stools, diarrhea, allergic reaction, those at risk for excessive bleeding, and those at risk of immune suppression.

5

OPTIMIZE CEREBRAL BLOOD FLOW

The adult brain weighs about two percent of the total body weight but typically receives 15% of the body's cardiac output to maintain function. Proper blood flow is closely regulated by body mechanisms to insure the brain's health and to meet its vital metabolic needs. Two important factors in regulating cerebral blood flow are the cerebral pressure and the diameter of cerebral blood vessels.

An increase in blood flow known as hyperemia can increase intracranial pressure. An increased intracranial pressure can compress and damage the delicate brain tissues. Increased intracranial pressure can be due to increased pressure in the brain tissues either by a tumor, bleeding into the brain or fluid on the brain. Aneurysm, stroke, brain tumor and traumatic head injury are causes of increased intracranial pressure.

Too little cerebral blood flow, much less common than hyperemia, is known as ischemia and can damage and ultimately cause cellular death to the affected brain cells. The brain can withstand a very short period without blood flow due to the constant need of oxygen to the brain cells which supply energy to the neurons. The constant blood flow also removes metabolic wastes from the cells. Without oxygen the brain suffers irreversible cellular injury within three to eight minutes under most circumstances.

After my TBI, I was diagnosed with fluid on my brain or brain edema. Though my initial injury was considered minor the fluid caused an increase in pressure on my brain. My fall caused traumatic shearing affects to the neurons of my brain initially but the brain swelling and increased pressure caused ongoing damage. Increased intracranial pressure is a serious and potentially deadly consequence many of us with brain injuries, whether traumatic or ischemic have faced. Increasing blood flow without increasing cranial pressure is an important aspect of improved cognitive and executive function.

After my TBI I was given a stimulant to increase my ability to mentally process, an attempt to strive for normal brain functioning. I have met many survivors who are also reliant on stimulants whether prescribed by their physicians or are self-prescribing as in drinking caffeinated beverages.

Caffeine, a neurostimulant, is used by many as a source of energy and to aid in focused thinking. While caffeine will give you a boost of energy and can help focus your thinking it is a vasoconstrictor and limits cerebral blood flow.

Think of water running through a garden hose. If you put your thumb over the end of the hose the water starts to squirt out. The water pressure has increased because your thumb has constricted the size of the opening that the water leaves the hose. Caffeine has the same effect on your brain's blood vessels. It increases the intracranial pressure by constricting the brain's blood flow.

In my case, use of a stimulant got me up and moving; it aided my ability to focus, but caused serious side effects. I suffered high blood pressure, anxiety, irritability and sleep disturbances. My days became vicious cycles of frenetic energy with sluggish lethargic collapses. My brain and body were paying a terrible price for functionality. I soon found myself in need of anti-anxiety, hypertensive and insomnia medication to combat the effects of the stimulant. I questioned the sense of it.

Decreased cerebral blood flow can happen instantaneously after brain injury and its effects can be long lasting. Progressive declines in cerebral blood are associated with aging and some neurodegenerative conditions.

Research has shown that gingko biloba can increase cerebral blood flow. Gingko biloba at 60mg taken twice a day showed improved cerebral blood flow in just four weeks. Gingko biloba is being researched further for potential efficacy in dementia and Alzheimer's disease. A research review of Alzheimer's sufferers showed benefits in activities of daily living and cognition at 240 mg a day.

6

ANTIOXIDANTS

Antioxidants are substances that protect cells from damage and the harmful effects of unstable molecules known as free radicals. Free radicals damage cells leading to a change in cells morphology or cellular structure and its function. This damage can cause cell death. Changes in cell size, shape and functionality may also lead to cancer.

Some of our vitamins are also antioxidants. Vitamins A, C and E function as protectors of other cells and are considered antioxidants. Other popular antioxidants are beta-carotene, lutein and selenium.

Alpha-lipoic acid is a strong antioxidant, anti-inflammatory and neuroprotectant. Alpha-lipoic acid helps protect the functioning of the blood brain barrier and in alleviating brain edema (see Chapter 5). The blood brain barrier physiologically

41

functions to protect the brain from some substances (drugs) while letting other pass freely into the brain.

Studies show that Alpha-lipoic acid helped reverse biochemical alterations in brain tissue in mice that were TBI induced. Lipoic acid is both safe and effective in short and long term studies in neutralizing and lowering the effects of oxidative stress on the brain, which are triggered after TBI.

Curcumin found in the Indian spice turmeric is in the ginger family. Curcumin is a powerful antioxidant that counteracts the effects of oxidative stress and synaptic plasticity after TBI. Curcumin enhances cognition post TBI. Exciting research shows curcumin in combination with vitamin D3 may inhibit the buildup of beta-amyloid plaques like those seen in Alzheimer's disease. Along with curcumin's powerful neuroprotective effects it can also boost brain-derived neurotropic factor, benefitting normal brain function and recovery following brain insults.

Since curcumin is readily available, it is easy to add to your diet. For improved absorption I recommend using curcumin with black pepper. Peperine derived from black pepper increases the bioavailability of curcumin with no adverse effects. Using a spoon add some olive oil, a teaspoon of curcumin and some freshly ground black pepper, mix and swallow.

Glutathione is another powerful and brain healthy antioxidant. Traumatic brain injury causes brain energy depletion and decreases levels of glutathione. Research has shown that glutathione reduces the adverse effects of oxidative stress on the brain following brain injury and promotes neuron repair.

Glutathione cannot be absorbed directly but it is made in the body. The best method to insure adequate glutathione levels is to eat a healthy balanced diet and exercise. If you wish to boost your glutathione levels further adding the following supplements to your regime N-acetyl cysteine (NAC), milk thistle and S-Adenosyl-Methionine (SAMe) will be beneficial.

7

HYDRATION

Water makes up 75% of the human body and about 85% of the brain. Experts believe that three quarters of the United States' population is suffering from chronic dehydration.

Water transports nutrients, allows our digestive system to produce enzymes, improve transit time to rid us of waste, maintain cell structure, lubricate joints, maintain body temperature, control blood pressure and transport neurotransmitters which effect sleep, mood and behavior. It's important!

<u>Try this simple exercise:</u>

1. Calculate the number of ounces of water you drink in a day (one cup = 8 ounces)   _____

2. Subtract the amount (in ounces) of caffeine you drink in a day   (-) _____

3. Subtract any alcoholic beverages (in ounces)

you consumed today*   (-) _____

4. Equals your water consumption for one day (in ounces)   _____

If less than 64 ounces and this is fairly typical for you, YOU ARE DEHYDRATED. You should be consuming at least eight 8-ounce glasses of water or non-caffeinated herbal tea every day.

*If you are a survivor and are consuming alcohol I recommend you reread Chapter 1 and find out why you <u>feel</u> you need it.

A rule I use for my clients; *only water or herbal (non-caffeine) teas count toward your eight glasses a day.* Juice, lemonade, diet sodas or any drink that is mixed or contains sugar, I consider a food. If you exercise, sweat, take a prescribed stimulant (common medication after brain injury) or take a diuretic (a type of blood pressure pill) then you will need to drink more than 64 total ounces a day.

For the longest time after my injury food had little or no taste. Most of what I drank had to be very sweet for me to taste it. Many brain injury survivors have memory issues; difficulty with their taste receptors; or feel they need the stimulatory effect of caffeine. This may be true but you also need water. Try to start drinking water, limit caffeine, and over time get up to eight-8 ounce glasses a day.

When you begin to drink more you will urinate more frequently. For this reason try to drink your daily intake of water three or more hours before you go to bed. Also, help yourself succeed...fill two quart jars with water and have them sitting around your house. If you see it you're more prone to drink it.

But I just don't get thirsty! I know, I was there too after my injury but your body still needs the water to function. Exercise triggered my thirst. Keep working at it, I know you can do it!

I am now a fan of green tea. Green tea does contain some caffeine but only a portion of the caffeine content that a cup of coffee contains. It is not enough to increase heart rate and therefore has a mild stimulatory effect on the central nervous system. Plus green tea contains flavonoids and polyphenols, which supply health benefits to the body.

Green tea has been shown to improve memory and attention in mild cognitive impairment. Green tea benefits were shown at two cups a day but higher consumption of green tea is associated with lower prevalence of cognitive impairment in humans.

Green tea polyphenols have been shown to improve cognitive performance induced by psychological stressors. Think of the polyphenols in green tea as natural *mood food* protecting against cognitive and psychiatric disorders.

The polyphenols in green tea and curcumin are showing significant benefits in the therapeutic intervention of anxiety and depression. Also, the polyphenols in green tea have been combined with caffeine, as in some weight loss products, which do create a thermogenic (fat burning) effect on the body.

8

NEUROTRANSMITTERS

Neurotransmitters are chemicals released by nerve cells to signal or communicate other nerve cells to allow the nerve cells to function in an expected fashion. Brain injury can damage the brain's ability to make sufficient amounts of the neurotransmitters needed and can also damage the nerve cells ability to receive the signals adequately.

Acetylcholine (Ach) is a neurotransmitter in the peripheral and central nervous system (cholinergic system). It is inhibitory on the central nervous system, first being identified in cardiac muscle where it slows the heart rate.

Acetylcholine is a neuromodulator with effects on brain plasticity, attention, memory and our reward system (why we want to do things). It also promotes rapid eye movement sleep (REM). Sleep is important to solidify newly learned thoughts and to allow recall of that information at a future time (See Figure 7).

If you are a brain injury survivor do you remember how tired you were early in your recovery? Maybe you still are. Fatigue, sleepiness and insomnia are troublesome consequences of brain injury. Early after my injury I could have slept constantly but as my awareness improved my ability to find comfort in a good night's sleep diminished. Many survivors suffer insomnia which has a negative impact on your relationships with others, on your feelings, and on your quality of life. Insomnia can directly relate to your chances of developing depression.

The following supplements have been shown to improve your body's ability to make acetylcholine. N-Acetyl-Cysteine (NAC), L-carnitine, Taurine, gingko biloba and vitamins B1, B5 and B12. Phosphatidyl choline is a precursor to acetylcholine and research has shown that phophatidylcholine used in conjunction with vitamin B12 increased acetylcholine concentrations and improved memory acquisition and retention.

Dopamine is a neurotransmitter produced in the body and active in the brain. The human brain has at least five types of dopamine receptors. Dopamine is responsible for reward-driven learning. Highly addictive stimulatory drugs, such as cocaine and methamphetamine have direct activity on the dopamine system. Outgoing people vs. introverts are suspected as having greater dopamine production.

Dopamine is also used to create other neurotransmitters in the body. Therefore, a decrease in dopamine can affect other functioning aspects of the brain. It is believed that disruption of the dopamine pathways of the brain after brain injury can have a profound effect on the cascade of symptoms a survivor can exhibit. Therapies targeting dopamine have consistently shown benefits in attention, improved behavioral outcome, problem solving, executive function and memory.

Dopamine cannot be taken orally since it will not cross the blood brain barrier. L-Phenylalanine, L-Tyrosine and L-Dopa are amino acids that the body uses to synthesize dopamine; they are normally consumed in our diet.

GABA, known as gamma- aminobutyric acid, is the main inhibitory neurotransmitter in our central nervous system. GABA reduces excessive brain activity and has the ability to instill a sense of calm. GABA can improve sleep quality and ease pain. It aids in production of endorphins which can give you a sense of well being. GABA is highly concentrated in the hypothalamus and hippocampus.

The hypothalamus controls body temperature, thirst, hunger, emotional responses and sexual behavior. It also controls hormone production of the pituitary gland and our circadian rhythm; sleep and wake cycles. The hippocampus, part of the limbic system, plays a part in three main areas; long term memory, space and inhibition.

A deficiency of GABA can lead to irritability, restlessness and anxiety. GABA deficiency is suspected in working memory deficits. GABA inhibits the firing of your brain cells. Extended excitability and firing of brain cells is suspected in seizures.   GABA is believed to inhibit post-traumatic epilepsy.

Current research is conflicting about GABA use early after TBI.   Citrus, beef liver, broccoli and halibut increase glutamic acid and glutamate. Glutamic acid and glutamate are precursors to glutamine.   Whole grains, brown rice and oats increase glutamine.   Glutamine is a precursor to GABA.   GABA can also be increased naturally by doing yoga.   Those receiving medically supervised GABA treatments may experience slight tingling and increased heart rate during initial dosing.

5-Hydroxytryptophan (5-HTP) is an amino acid and a precursor for the production of very important neurotransmitters; Serotonin, Melatonin and Tryptophan, which control our daily functioning through our circadian rhythms.   5-HTP has been reported to have a beneficial effect on sleep, mood, anxiety, appetite, and pain sensation.

ACETYLCHOLINE (Ach)	Attention
	Memory
	Reward system
DOPAMINE	Attention
	Behavior
	Executive function
	Memory
GAMMA-AMINOBUTRYIC ACID (GABA)	Improve sleep
	Ease pain
5-HYDROXYTRYPTOPHAN (5-HTP)	Improve sleep
	Mood
	Appetite
	Lessen anxiety
	Ease pain

Figure 7. Neurotransmitter functions.

A Final Word

I have used all of these strategies at one time or another during my recovery. I find my exercise routine to be rejuvenating. It's my "reset" button if I'm having a bad day, A nice walk or a few minutes of yoga can refocus me mentally and help calm my anxiety.

I started out doing balance exercises on a Wii™. I couldn't stand on one leg without holding on to a chair. Eventually, I was able to ride a bike again. I went for a nice long ride one afternoon only to forget that it was going to get dark. Seriously, I think back in amazement, *I was really that bad cognitively; that I didn't remember it was going to get dark*? That that happened still astounds me.

I want you to do some soul searching and ask yourself how much do you value your health and feeling good? Your injury took something from you; health, respect, friends, spouse, your job? I know it's hard, I know you're hurting. Are you eager to feel better, to lose weight, to have more energy? If so, it's time for change, time for you to be more proactive in your health care.

It takes great perseverance to regain your health and an enormous amount of compassion to accept yourself.

Change is never easy but if you make positive lifestyle changes you will benefit. I wish you the best of luck on your own brain health journey!

Susan M. Plank, D.C.

RESOURCES

Weight-control Information Network
http://win.niddk.nih.gov/publications/PDFs/Changing_Your_Habits.pdf
Weight loss information provided by National Institutes of Diabetes and Digestive and Kidney Disease (NIDDK).

Active
active.com/fitness/calculators/body fat
Active offers resources on getting fit and staying active. It also offers a calculator for you to be able to compute your percent body fat.

American Institute for Cancer Research
aicr.org
AICR offers an interactive website offering BMI calculation, weight loss tips and healthy recipes.

My Fitness Pal
myfitnesspal.com
An interactive website that allows you to track your wellness goals; enter the foods you eat, exercise and water consumption and the website will calculate your total calories. I use this with my own clients.

Brain Injury Association of America

biausa.org

This website is an informational and advocacy site and can direct you to your state brain injury association.

Lumosity

lumosity.com

Lumosity is an interactive brain game website that can help you to improve your brain's health and performance.

Fit Brains

fitbrains.com

Fit brain provides fun brain fitness games to help improve brain function.

Brain Injury Survivor's Recommended Supplement List

	NAME	RDA	UNITS	FREQUENCY
MULTIVITAMIN	Multivitamin containing:			ONCE DAILY
	VITAMIN A	3000M* 2333 F	IU	
	VITAMIN A: 50% AS BETA-CAROTENE	2500	IU	
	B1, THIAMIN	1.2 M* 1.1 F	mg	
	B2, RIBOFLAVIN	1.3 M* 1.1 F	mg	
	B3, NIACIN	16 M* 14 F	mg	
	B6,PYRIDOXINE	1.3	mg	
	B12	2.4	mcg	
	FOLIC ACID/ FOLATE	400	mcg	
	VITAMIN C	90 M* 75 F	mg	
	VITAMIN D	600	IU	
	VITAMIN E	22.5	IU	

*M=MALE
F=FEMALE

Brain Injury Survivor's Recommended Supplement List (continued)

FATTY ACIDS	OMEGA-3	1000	mg	1-3 X/ DAY W FOOD
BLOOD FLOW	GINGKO BILOBA	60	mg	2-4 X/ DAY

ANTIOXIDANTS	ALPHA-LIPOIC ACID	100	mg	ONCE DAILY
	CURCUMIN (TURMERIC EXTRACT)	500	mg	1-2 X /DAY
	GLUTATHIONE*			
	N-ACETYL CYSTEINE (NAC)	200	mg	ONCE DAILY
	MILK THISTLE (SILYMARIN)	200	mg	ONCE DAILY
	S-ADENOSYL-METHIONINE (SAMe)	400	mg	ONCE DAILY

HYDRATE	WATER	8	oz	8 X/ DAY
	GREEN TEA (POLYPHENOLS)	8	oz	2 X/ DAY

References

Chapter 1   Making Good Choice: How to Change Your Habits

Gretchen L. Zimmerman, Psy.D, Cynthia G. Olsen, M.D., and Michael F. Bosworth,D.O. A 'Stages of Change' Approach to Helping Patients Change Behavior. *Am Fam Physician*. 2000 Mar 1;61(5):1409-1416.

National Institute on Alcohol Abuse and Alcoholism (NIAAA). US Dept of Health and Human Services. NIH study finds hospitalizations increase for alcohol and drug overdoses. *NIH News*. Tuesday, September 20, 2011.

National Institutes of Health. National Institute on Drug Abuse. The Science of Drug Abuse and Addiction. www.drugabuse.gov

David D. Burns,M.D., *The Feeling Good Handbook*

Siervo M, Nasti G, Stephan BC, Papa A, Muscariello E, Wells JC, Prado CM, Colantuoni A. Effects of intentional weight loss on physical and cognitive function in middle-aged and older obese participants: a pilot study. J Am Coll Nutr. 2012 Apr;31(2):79-86.

D'Anci KE, Watts KL, Appetite. Kanarek RB, Taylor HA. Low-carbohydrate weight-loss diets. Effects on cognition and mood. *Appetite*. 2009 Feb;52(1):96-103. Epub 2008 Aug 29.

Siervo M, Arnold R, Wells JC, Tagliabue A, Colantuoni A, Albanese E, Brayne C, Stephan BC. Intentional weight loss in overweight and obese individuals and cognitive function: a systematic review and meta-analysis. *Obes Rev*. 2011 Nov;12(11):968-83. doi: 10.1111/j.1467-789X.2011.00903.x. Epub 2011 Jul 18.

Jourdan C, Brugel D, Hubeaux K, Toure H, Laurent-Vannier A, Chevignard M. Weight gain after childhood traumatic brain injury: a matter of concern. *Dev Med Child Neurol*. 2012 Jul;54(7):624-8. doi: 10.1111/j.1469-8749.2012.04291.x. Epub 2012 Apr 24.

Ashrafian H. Henry VIII's obesity following traumatic brain injury. *Endocrine*. 2012 Aug;42(1):218-9.

Elias MF, Goodell AL, Waldstein SR. Obesity, cognitive functioning and dementia: back to the future. *J Alzheimers Dis*. 2012;30 Suppl 2:S113-25.

M F Elias , P K Elias, L M Sullivan, P A Wolf and R B D'Agostino Lower cognitive function in the presence of obesity and hypertension: the Framingham heart study. *International Journal of Obesity* (2003) 27, 260–268. doi:10.1038/sj.ijo.802225

Casanueva FF, Leal A, Koltowska-Häggström M, Jonsson P, Góth MI. Traumatic brain injury as a relevant cause of growth hormone deficiency in adults: A KIMS-based study. *Arch Phys Med Rehabil.* 2005 Mar;86(3):463-8.

Daviglus ML, Bell CC, Berrettini W, Bowen PE, Connolly ES, Cox NJ, Dunbar-Jacob JM, Granieri EC, Hunt G, McGarry K, Patel D, Potosky AL, Sanders-Bush E, Silberberg D, Trevisan M. National Institutes of Health State-of-the-Science Conference Statement: Preventing Alzheimer's Disease and Cognitive Decline. *NIH Consens State Sci Statements.* 2010 Apr 26–28;27(4):1–30.

Medic-Stojanoska M, Pekic S, Curic N, Djilas-Ivanovic D, Popovic V. Evolving hypopituitarism as a consequence of traumatic brain injury (TBI) in childhood - call for attention. *Endocrine.* 2007 Jun;31(3):268-71.

Popovic V. GH deficiency as the most common pituitary defect after TBI: clinical implications. *Pituitary.* 2005;8(3-4):239-43.

Chapter 3   High Potency Multivitamin

Tucker KL, Qiao N, Scott T, Rosenberg I, Spiro A 3rd. High homocysteine and low B vitamins predict cognitive decline in aging men: the Veterans Affairs Normative Aging Study. *Am J Clin Nutr.* 2005 Sep;82(3):627-35.

Kennedy DO, Haskell CF. Vitamins and cognition: what is the evidence? *Drugs.* 2011 Oct 22;71(15):1957-71. doi: 10.2165/11594130-000000000-00000.

Grima NA, Pase MP, Macpherson H, Pipingas A. The effects of multivitamins on cognitive performance: a systematic review and meta-analysis. *J Alzheimers Dis.* 2012;29(3):561-9.

Chapter 4   Fatty Acids and Fish Oil

Robinson JG, Ijioma N, Harris W. Omega-3 fatty acids and cognitive function in women. *Womens Health (Lond Engl).* 2010 Jan;6(1):119-34.

Kidd PM. Omega-3 DHA and EPA for cognition, behavior, and mood: clinical findings and structural-functional synergies with cell membrane phospholipids. *Altern Med Rev.* 2007 Sep;12(3):207-27.

Hooijmans CR, Pasker-de Jong PC, de Vries RB, Ritskes-Hoitinga M. The effects of long-term omega-3 fatty acid supplementation on cognition and Alzheimer's pathology in animal models of Alzheimer's disease: a systematic review and meta-analysis. *J Alzheimers Dis*. 2012;28(1):191-209.

Barringer N, Conkright W. Omega-3 Fatty Acid Ingestion as a TBI Prophylactic. *J Spec Oper Med*. 2012 Fall;12(3):5-7.

Shin SS, Dixon CE. Oral fish oil restores striatal dopamine release after traumatic brain injury. *Neurosci Lett*. 2011 Jun 8;496(3):168-71. Epub 2011 Apr 14.

Chapter 5   Optimize Cerebral Blood Flow

Hill, Dr. Lisa, Royal Oldham Hospital, UK, Cerebral Blood Flow and Intracranial Pressure

Ling GSF. Traumatic brain injury and spinal cord injury. In: Goldman L, Ausiello D, eds. *Cecil Medicine* . 23rd ed. Philadelphia, Pa: Saunders Elsevier; 2007: chap 422.

Rosenberg GA. Brain edema and disorders of cerebrospinal fluid circulation. In: Bradley WG, Daroff RB, Fenichel GM, Jankovic J, eds. *Bradley: Neurology in Clinical Practice*. 5th ed. Philadelphia, Pa: Butterworth-Heinemann Elsevier; 2008:chap 63.

Kochanek PM, Hendrich KS, Dixon CE, Schiding JK, Williams DS, Ho C. Cerebral blood flow at one year after controlled cortical impact in rats: assessment by magnetic resonance imaging. *Journal of Neurotrauma*. 2002 Sep;19(9):1029-37.

Mashayekh A, Pham DL, Yousem DM, Dizon M, Barker PB, Lin DD. Effects of Ginkgo biloba on cerebral blood flow assessed by quantitative MR perfusion imaging: a pilot study. *Neuroradiology*. 2011 Mar;53(3):185-91.

Janssen IM, Sturtz S, Skipka G, Zentner A, Velasco Garrido M, Busse R. Ginkgo biloba in Alzheimer's disease: a systematic review. *Wien Med Wochenschr*. 2010 Dec;160(21-22):539-46.

Chapter 6   Antioxidants

John M. Ringman, Sally A. Frautschy,[2] Gregory M. Cole, Donna L. Masterman, and Jeffrey L. Cummings ,A Potential Role of the Curry Spice Curcumin in Alzheimer's Disease. *Curr Alzheimer Res. 2005 April; 2(2): 131–136.*

Suzhen Dong, Qingwen Zeng, E. Siobhan Mitchell, Jin Xiu, Yale Duan, Chunxia Li, Jyoti K. Tiwari, Yinghe Hu, Xiaohua Cao, and Zheng Zhao, Cumin Enhances Neurogenesis and Cognition in Aged Rats: Implications for Transcriptional Interactions Related to Growth and Synaptic Plasticity. *PLoS One*. 2012; 7(2): e31211. Published online 2012 February 16. doi: 10.1371/journal.pone.0031211

Gomez-Pinilla F. Collaborative effects of diet and exercise on cognitive enhancement. *Nutrition Health.* 2011;20(3-4):165-9.

Shoba G, Joy D, Joseph T, Majeed M, Rajendran R, Srinivas PS. Influence of piperine on the pharmacokinetics of curcumin in animals and human volunteers. *Planta Med.* 1998 May;64(4):353-6.

Khan M, Sakakima H, Dhammu TS, Shunmugavel A, Im YB, Gilg AG, Singh AK, Singh I. S-nitrosoglutathione reduces oxidative injury and promotes mechanisms of neurorepair following traumatic brain injury in rats. *Journal Neuroinflammation.* 2011 Jul 6;8:78.

Prieto R, Tavazzi B, Taya K, Barrios L, Amorini AM, Di Pietro V, Pascual JM, Marmarou A, Marmarou CR. Brain energy depletion in a rodent model of diffuse traumatic brain injury is not prevented with administration of sodium lactate. *Brain Res.* 2011 Aug 2;1404:39-49. Epub 2011 Jun 12

Chapter 7   Hydration

Fernando Gomez-Pinilla and Trang T J Nguyen · Natural mood foods: The actions of polyphenols against psychiatric and cognitive disorders. *Nutr Neurosci.* 2012 May; 15(3): 127–133.

Park SK, Jung IC, Lee WK, Lee YS, Park HK, Go HJ, Kim K, Lim NK, Hong JT, Ly SY, Rho SS. A combination of green tea extract and l-theanine improves memory and attention in subjects with mild cognitive impairment: a double-blind placebo-controlled study. *J Med Food.* 2011 Apr;14(4):334-43. Epub 2011 Feb 8.

Chen WQ, Zhao XL, Hou Y, Li ST, Hong Y, Wang DL, Cheng YY. Protective effects of green tea polyphenols on cognitive impairments induced by psychological stress in rats. *Behav Brain Res.* 2009 Aug 24;202(1):71-6. Epub 2009 Mar 21.

Kuriyama S, Hozawa A, Ohmori K, Shimazu T, Matsui T, Ebihara S, Awata S, Nagatomi R, Arai H, Tsuji I. Green tea consumption and cognitive function: a cross-sectional study from the Tsurugaya Project 1. *Am J Clin Nutr.* 2006 Feb;83(2):355-61.

Gisele Pereira Dias, Nicole Cavegn, Alina Nix, Mário Cesar do Nascimento Bevilaqua, Doris Stangl, Muhammad Syahrul Anwar Zainuddin, Antonio Egidio Nardi, Patricia Franca Gardino, and Sandrine Thuret. The Role of Dietary Polyphenols on Adult Hippocampal Neurogenesis: Molecular Mechanisms and Behavioural Effects on Depression and Anxiety. *Oxid Med Cell Longev.* 2012; 2012: 541971.

Quideau S, Deffieux D, Douat-Casassus C, Pouységu L. Plant polyphenols: chemical properties, biological activities, and synthesis. *Angew Chem Int* Ed Engl. 2011;50:586–621

Manach C, Scalbert A, Morand C, Rémésy C, Jiménez L. Polyphenols: food sources and bioavailability. *Am J Clin Nutr.* 2004;79:727–47.

Chapter 8   Neurotransmitters

Cantor JB, Bushnik T, Cicerone K, Dijkers MP, Gordon W, Hammond FM, Kolakowsky-Hayner SA, Lequerica A, Nguyen M, Spielman LA. Insomnia, Fatigue, and Sleepiness in the First 2 Years After Traumatic Brain Injury: An NIDRR TBI Model System Module Study. *J Head Trauma Rehabil.* 2012 Nov;27(6):E1-E14.

Lyeth BG, Hayes RL. Cholinergic and opioid mediation of traumatic brain injury. *J Neurotrauma.* 1992 May;9 Suppl 2:S463-74.

Angst J, Woggon B, Schoepf J. The treatment of depression with L-5-hydroxytryptophan versus imipramine. Results of two open and one double-blind study. *Arch Psychiatr Nervenkr.* 1977;224:175â€"186.

Attele AS, Xie JT, Yuan CS. Treatment of insomnia: an alternative approach.*Altern Med Rev.* 2000;5(3):249-259.

Birdsall TC. 5-Hydroxytryptophan: a clinically-effective serotonin precursor. *Altern Med Rev.* 1998;3:271â€"280.

Byerley WF, et al. 5-Hydroxytryptophan: a review of its antidepressant efficacy and adverse effects. *J Clin Psychopharmacol.* 1987;7:127-137.

Cangiano C, et al. Effects of oral 5-hydroxy-tryptophan on energy intake and macronutrient selection in non-insulin dependent diabetic patients. *Int J Obes Relat Metab Disord.* 1998; 22:648-654.

Cangiano C, Ceci F, Cascino A, et al. Eating behavior and adherence to dietary prescriptions in obese adult subjects treated with 5-hydroxytryptophan. *J Clin Nutr.* 1992;56:863-867.

Caruso I, Sarzi Puttini P, Cazzola M, et al. Double-blind study of 5-hydroxytryptophan versus placebo in the treatment of primary fibromyalgia syndrome. *J Int Med Res.* 1990;18:201-209.

Cauffield JS, Forbes HJ. Dietary supplements used in the treatment of depression, anxiety, and sleep disorders. *Lippincotts Prim Care Pract.* 1999; 3(3):290-304.

Ceci F, Cangiano C, Cairella M, Cascino A, et al. The effects of oral 5-hydroxytryptophan administration on feeding behavior in obese adult female subjects. *J Neural Transm.* 1989;76:109-117.

Curcio JJ, Kim LS, Wollner D, Pockaj BA. The potential of 5-hydryxtryptophan for hot flash reduction: a hypothesis. *Altern Med Rev.* 2005;10(3):216-21.

DeBenedittis G, Massei R. Serotonin precursors in chronic primary headache. A double-blind cross-over study with L-5-hydroxytryptophan vs. placebo. *J Neurosurg Sci*. 1985; 29:239-248.

Elko CJ, Burgess JL, Robertson WO. Zolpidem-associated hallucinations and serotonin reuptake inhibition: a possible interaction. *J Toxicol Clin Toxicol*. 1998;36(3):195-203.

Freedman RR. Treatment of menopausal hot flashes with 5-hydroxytryptophan. *Maturitas*. 2010 Apr;65(4):383-5.

Gardner DM, Lynd LD. Sumatriptan contraindications and the serotonin syndrome. *Ann Pharmacother*. 1998;32(1):33-38.

Iovieno N, Dalton ED, Fava M, Mischoulon D. Second-tier natural antidepressants: Review and critique. *J Affect Disord*. 2010 Jun 24.

Joffe RT, Sokolov ST. Co-administration of fluoxetine and sumatriptan: the Canadian experience. *Acta Psychiatr Scand*. 1997;95(6):551-552.

Joly P, Lampert A, Thomine E, Lauret P. Development of pseudobullous morphea and sclero-derma-like illness during therapy with L-5-hydroxytryptophan and carbidopa. *J Am Acad Dermatol*. 1991;25(2):332-333.

Juhl JH. Primary fibromyalgia syndrome and 5-hydroxy-L-tryptophan: a 90-day open study. *Altern Med Rev*. 1998;3:367-375.

Mason BJ, Blackburn KH. Possible serotonin syndrome associated with tramadol and sertraline coadministration. *Ann Pharmacother*. 1997;31(2):175-177.

Meyers S. Use of neurotransmitter precursors for treatment of depression. *Altern Med Rev*. 2000;5(1):64-71.

Perry NK. Venlafaxine-induced serotonin syndrome with relapse following amitripyline. *Postgrad Med J*. 2000;76(894):254.

Puttini PS, Caruso I. Primary fibromyalgia and 5-hydroxy-L-tryptophan: a 90-day open study. *J Int Med Res*. 1992;20:182-189.

Rakel D. *Rakel Integrative Medicine, 2nd ed*. Philadelphia, PA: Saunders; 2008;47.

Reibring L, Agren H, Hartvig P, et al. Uptake and utilization of [beta-11c] 5-hydroxytryptophan (5-HTP) in human brain studied by positron emission tomography. *Pyschiatry Research*. 1992;45:215-225.

Ribeiro CA. L-5-Hydroxytryptophan in the prophylaxis of chronic tension-type headache: a double-blind, randomized, placebo-controlled study. *Headache*. 2000 Jun;40(6):451-6.

Shaw K, Turner J, Del Mar C. Are tryptophan and 5-hydroxytryptophan effective treatments for depression? A meta-analysis. *Aust N Z J Psychiatry*. 2002 Aug;36(4):488-91.

Sternberg EM, Van Woert MH, Young SN, et al. Development of a scleroderma-like illness during therapy with L-5-

hydroxytryptophan and carbidopa. *New Eng J Med*. 1980;303:782-787.

Toner LC, Tsambiras BM, Catalano G, et al. Central nervous system side effects associated with zolpidem treatment. *Clin Neuropharmacol*. 2000;23(1):54-58.

Van Praag HM. Management of depression with serotonin precursors. *Biol Psychiatry*. 1981;16:291-310.

Zmilacher K, et al. L-5-hydroxytryptophan alone and in combination with a peripheral decarboxylase inhibitor in the treatment of depression. *Neuropsychobiology*. 1988;20:28–33.

http://www.neuroanatomy.wisc.edu/coursebook/neuro2(2).pdf

http://neuroscienceupdate.cumc.columbia.edu/popups/pdfs/PeterCarmel.pdf

http://vanat.cvm.umn.edu/NeuroLectPDFs/LectDienceph.pdf

Dr Ananya Mandal, MD. *News-Medical*. What is the Hypothalamus? November 27, 2012

www.ingramcontent.com/pod-product-compliance
Lightning Source LLC
Chambersburg PA
CBHW071623170526

45166CB00003B/1164